D0292204

Aromatherapy oils, also known as "essential" or "volatile" oils, are the highly fragrant liquid components of aromatic plants, trees, and grasses. They can be found in different parts of the plant including the petals (rose), bark (cinnamon), resin (frankincense).

The term "aromatherapy" dates back to the 1920s when French cosmetic chemist René-Maurice Gattefossé discovered the healing properties of essential oils.

He suffered severe burns to his hand in a laboratory explosion and treated the wound with undiluted lavender essence. It healed without a scar. Essential oils were found to contain powerful antiseptic and painkilling properties.

At that time, Italian doctors, Gatti and Cajola, demonstrated the therapeutic effects of smelling essential oils. The holistic usage of essential oils was further developed in the 1950s when Austrian-born Marguerite Maury introduced the idea of combining them with massage.

Aromatics through the Ages

The true founders of aromatherapy are thought to be the ancient Egyptians. They extracted aromatic oils from exotic flowers by squeezing the oil from the petals. The preservative powers of the oils made them an essential part of the embalming process, and they were also blended into perfumes and used as incense.

The Greeks advocated the wearing of fragrant flower garlands and of taking daily aromatic baths, and soon the Romans too were extolling the virtues of healing balms and aromatherapy massage.

Persian physician Avicenna
believed that plant essences
strengthened body and spirit,
and the Persians developed a
passion for the perfume derived
from the essential oil of
red roses.

In ancient China, Chinese
alchemists believed that plant
extracts contained magical
forces to help them develop the
elixir of life!

In the Mood

**Knowing a little about the
origins** of essential oils, you'll be keen to
practice the ancient art of aromatherapy for
yourself. It's the perfect way to achieve peace of
mind—think of it as nature's antidote to stress!

Create your own calming space by using incense
sticks or cones to scent your room. Candles
complement the theme—especially when they are
scented. Specially designed holders should be
used for both candles and incense.

Why not make your own aromatic candle? It's best to buy a chunky beeswax candle to give you the added benefit of honeyed scent! Light it and wait for the wax around the wick to melt. Then blow it out and carefully add a few drops of the essential oil to the molten wax BEFORE relighting.

Warning

Essential oils are highly flammable so NEVER add the oil while the candle is burning.

At the end of a long day, prepare to kick off your shoes and slide into a warm fragrant bath. This is an excellent way to indulge in essential oils as you'll absorb the oils through your nose and skin.

❁ Blend 2 ounces of carrier oil with 20 drops of your favorite smelling essential oil
❁ Store in an amber or cobalt glass bottle
❁ Run the bath first (otherwise the vapor will evaporate before you get in)
❁ Sprinkle 6 drops of oil on to the water's surface and agitate to disperse well
❁ Immerse yourself in heavenly scent!

Warning

Essential oils enter the bloodstream through the skin. NEVER apply them directly to your skin as they can be extremely potent. Dilute in a carrier oil and ALWAYS do a patch test first.

Patch test:

- ❁ Mix one drop of the essential oil into a teaspoon of carrier oil
- ❁ Rub a little of the mixture on the inside of your wrist
- ❁ Leave uncovered and unwashed for 24 hours
- ❁ If you suffer no redness or itching the oil is safe to use in a diluted form

Treat your partner to an aromatherapy massage—it will arouse the most primitive senses of smell and touch. Diluted in a carrier oil, then massaged into the skin, essential oils are sure to give the desired spine-tingling effect.

Make your own massage oil by mixing 8-10 drops of skin-friendly essential oil to 1 ounce of carrier oil. Try blending 2 drops of rose otto with 5 drops of sandalwood for a truly sensuous massage.

Tip!

For a superior quality massage, seek "unrefined" carrier oils that still contain their natural vitamins and skin enriching minerals.

Oil burners and incense cones are a wonderful way to bring harmony into your home.

- ✿ Simply pour some water into the reservoir (this will prevent the oil from heating too quickly)
- ✿ Add some drops of your preferred essential oil
- ✿ Light a candle and place underneath to heat the reservoir. As the water heats, the oil will gently warm through and your room will be redolent with gorgeous scent!
- ✿ Only ever light the incense cones on the ceramic dish provided with this set. Make sure it sits securely on top of a non-melting surface—never rest the dish on plastic
- ✿ Never touch the cones once lit and never leave them unattended

Fragranced Oils

Fragranced oils are not essential oils but they should be treated with the same care. They are usually designed to be used with an oil burner and are not for use on the skin.

After a bath or shower, your skin is warm and receptive and essential oils will be absorbed quickly. Make the most of it by treating yourself to a homemade massage oil that matches your skin type.

Warning

Remember the potency of these essential oils—patch test your skin before applying and NEVER apply undiluted.

Normal Skin

Mix 25 ml jojoba oil with 3 drops of lavender and 2 drops of neroli.

Dry Skin

Mix 25 ml peach kernal oil with 1 drop of chamomile, 4 drops of lavender, and 10 ml of avocado.

Sensitive Skin

Mix 30 ml almond oil with 1 drop of chamomile.

Oily Skin

Mix 25 ml jojoba oil with 3 drops of cedarwood and 2 drops of frankincense.

NOTE

5ml is equal to 1 teaspoon. Adjust accordingly.

Bed of Roses

The seductive power

of scent and the way in which it lifts our spirits is rooted deep within us—whether it's the smell of newly mown grass, the mouth-watering smell of baking in the kitchen, or the crisp clean fragrance of fresh laundry.

Bring a woody fragrance to your laundry by adding some drops of frankincense or sandalwood to the distilled water in your steam iron.

For restful sleep and sweet dreams mix 15 drops of rose otto or lavender oil to 125 ml of water and spray over your bed linen.

Keep drawers fresh by lining them with wallpaper that has first been cut to size and sprayed with a strong aromatic concentrate of your chosen essential oil (40 drops to 50 ml of water).

Tip!

If you have an open fire, perfume the room by burning aromatic plants such as lavender flowers and rosemary twigs.

Perfume notes were the creation of nineteenth century French perfumer Charles Piesse. He categorized the aroma of essential oils to relate to a scale of top, middle, and base notes, like those of a musical stave.

The perfume industry still uses these three categories today—a good blend of perfume is a well-balanced combination of top, middle, and base notes.

Tip!

Base notes "fix" the fragrance and make it last longer.

In aromatherapy, the top (head) notes are the most volatile essential oils because they are fast acting and evaporate quickly. Middle (heart) notes are therapeutic and balancing, and base (bottom) notes are the least volatile oils that have a long-lasting effect.

Stimulating your senses, the top note is what you smell first. This fades away leaving you with the heart note and when this too fades, you can still smell the bottom note which lingers long after the other two have gone.

Carrier oils (sometimes called vegetable, base, or fixed oils) are derived from the fatty portions of seeds, nuts, vegetables, and plants. These are the base oils used to dilute essential oils before applying them to the skin, so called because they "carry" the essential oil onto your skin.

Carrier oils do not evaporate when heated, neither do they impart their aroma as strongly as essential oils. For this reason always try to obtain "cold pressed" or "extra virgin" carrier oils as these will contain the most therapeutic properties.

Originating from the fatty portions of plants means that all carrier oils make excellent choices for massage as they are rich in nutrients and moisturizing properties.

Tip!

Purchase carrier oils in small quantities as their shelf life is only three months.

Apricot Kernel

Plant: Apricot Kernel

Botanical name: Prunus armeniaca

Origins: Extracted from the seed kernel of the fruit.

Aroma: Faint smell of marzipan.

Properties: Light textured, easily absorbed, contains vitamins A and C.

Uses: A special oil used mainly in beauty care, and an excellent base for a face or body massage.

Plant: Avocado

Botanical name: Persea americana

Origins: Best quality is cold pressed from the flesh of the fruit.

Aroma: Faintly nutty.

Properties: Highly penetrative, rich in essential fatty acids, betacarotene, and vitamin E.

Uses: A special oil used mainly in beauty care— excellent for dry, aging skin, or skin dehydrated by too much sunbathing!

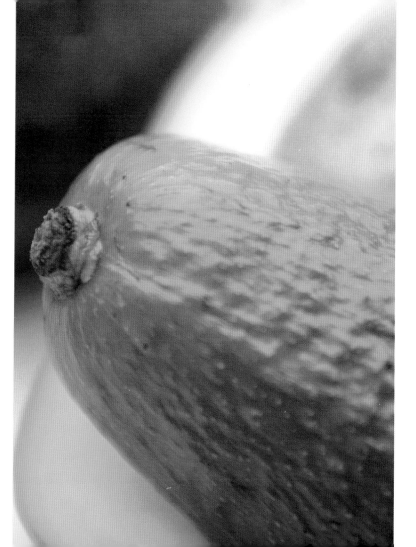

Borage

Plant: Borage

Botanical name: Borago officinalis

Origins: Warm pressed or solvent extracted from the tiny seeds of the beautiful blue starflower plant —is often labeled "Starflower" for this reason.

Aroma: Light and sweet.

Properties: Rich source of essential fatty acids.

Uses: A special oil used mainly in beauty care. The best way to enhance your skin is to take "Starflower" capsules as a nutritional supplement.

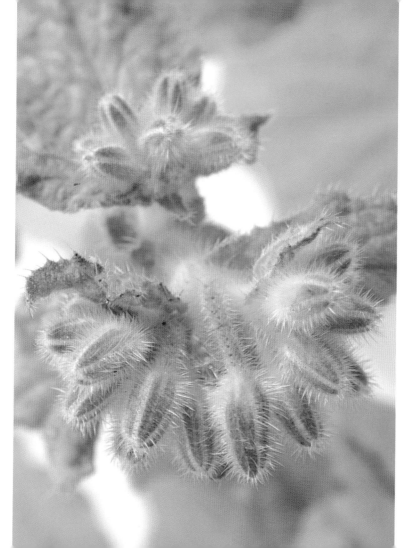

Plant: Evening Primrose

Botanical name: Oenothera biennis

Origins: Extracted from the tiny seeds of the bright yellow flowers which bloom only at night.

Aroma: Faint and musty.

Properties: Contains vitamins, minerals, and essential fatty acids.

Uses: A nutritional supplement to treat premenstrual syndrome, period pains, arthritis, and rheumatism. It is also excellent as a moisturizing beauty treatment.

Grapeseed

Plant: Grapeseed

Botanical name: Vitis vinifera

Origins: Heat extracted from the seeds of the fruit.

Aroma: Hardly any.

Properties: Heat extraction destroys the nutrients.

Uses: This is a popular massage oil.

Plant: Jojoba

Botanical name: Simmondsia chinensis

Origins: Liquid wax extracted from the beans of the plant.

Aroma: Hardly any.

Properties: Highly penetrative, also has some anti-inflammatory properties.

Uses: A special oil used mainly in beauty care. It is an excellent moisturizer for all skin types, and makes a good conditioning treatment for dry hair.

Plant: Peach Kernel

Botanical name: Prunus persica

Origins: Best quality is cold pressed from the kernels of the fruit.

Aroma: Delicate peachy aroma.

Properties: Fine textured so easily absorbed into the skin.

Uses: A special oil used mainly in beauty care, peach kernel oil is ideal for facial massage since it's kind to the skin. It will also add shine to hair.

Plant: Sweet Almond

Botanical name: Prunus dulcis

Origins: Extracted from the kernels of the sweet almond tree.

Aroma: Faint nutty scent.

Properties: Contains vitamins D and E, also has some anti-inflammatory properties.

Uses: It is excellent for treating psoriasis, eczema and dermatitis—or to relieve sunburn.

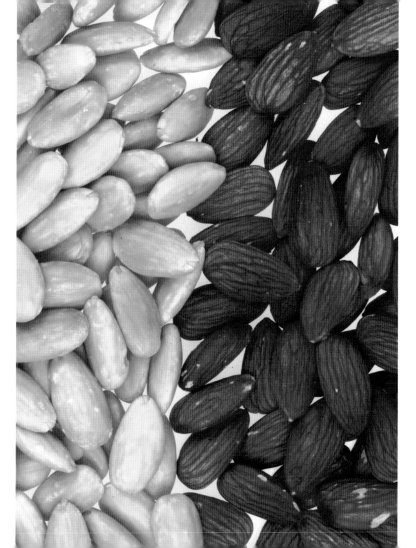

Infused Oils

Infused oils, sometimes called "macerated" oils, are commercially made when the amount of essential oil in the plant is very small and therefore expensive to extract. Fresh plant matter is soaked or "macerated" in a high quality carrier oil so that the essential oils are dissolved and impart their fragrance.

Plant: Hypericum (or St John's Wort)

Botanical name: Hypericum perforatum

Part used: Leaves and flowers.

Properties: Anti-inflammatory, anti-rheumatic.

Uses: It will ease rheumatism, sciatica, sunburn, and bruises.

Plant: Calendula (or marigold)

Botanical name: Calendula officinalis

Part used: Flowers.

Properties: Anti-inflammatory, antifungal.

Uses: This is excellent for treating eczema and diaper rash and soothes sore, inflamed, and itchy skin.

Now you know what constitutes
a carrier oil and what is meant
by an infused oil, you're ready
to try your hand at blending
and experimenting with some
aromatic oils of your choice!
Take your pick from the "Top
10" we've selected for you.
Don't forget to try composing
some subtle harmonies of your
own by blending some top,
middle, and base notes together
to compose a fragrant signature.

Chamomile

number 1

Plant: Chamomile

Botanical name: Anthemis nobilis

Origins: Extracted from the flower heads.

Aroma: Sweet and fruity.

Properties: Anti-inflammatory and antiseptic.

Uses: A good treatment for premenstrual syndrome, insect bites, stings, insomnia, and eczema.

Suggested Blends: Lavender, geranium, jasmine, rose otto, and neroli.

Perfume Note: Middle

WARNING!
Do NOT use if you are pregnant.

Plant: Cedarwood Atlas

Botanical name: Anthemis nobilis

Origins: Distilled from the wood shavings and sawdust.

Aroma: Sweet and woody.

Properties: Antiseptic, astringent, and sedative.

Uses: A good treatment for cystitis, fungal infections, dandruff, insect bites, and stings.

Suggested Blends: Frankincense, vetiver, and juniper.

Perfume Note: Base

number 2

Frankincense

number 3

Plant: Frankincense

Botanical name: Boswellia carterii

Origins: Extracted from the gum resin which collects when incisions are made into the bark.

Aroma: Warm and piney, with a hint of camphor.

Properties: Astringent, antiseptic, and sedative.

Uses: A good treatment for abscesses, ulcer's, asthma, and bronchitis.

Suggested Blends: Patchouli, rose otto, and juniper.

Perfume Note: Base

Geranium

number 4

Plant: Geranium

Botanical name: Pelargonium odoratissimum

Origins: Distilled from the leaves, stalks, and flowers

Aroma: Rose-scented, sweet, and heavy.

Properties: Analgesic, antiseptic, and astringent.

Uses: An excellent treatment for premenstrual syndrome, stress, cuts, and skin problems.

Suggested Blends: Lavender, and neroli.

Perfume Note: Middle

Lavender

Plant: Lavender

Botanical name: Lavandula augustifolia

Origins: Distilled from the flowering shrub tips.

Aroma: Sweet, flowery, and herbaceous.

Properties: Analgesic, sedative, and antiseptic.

Uses: Nature's first aid treatment for burns because it accelerates cell growth and repair. It has remarkable healing properties and can be used to alleviate high blood pressure and stress.

Suggested Blends: Rose otto, geranium, patchouli, and frankincense.

Perfume Note: Top/Middle

Mandarin

number 6

Plant: Mandarin

Botanical name: Citrus nobilis

Origins: Extracted from the peel of the fruit.

Aroma: Sweet and citrus.

Properties: Digestive, laxative, and sedative.

Uses: This is good for children's problems such as colic, hiccups, and coughs. It will also help to prevent stretch marks during pregnancy.

Suggested Blends: Lemongrass and rose otto.

Perfume Note: Top

Neroli

Plant: Neroli

Botanical name: Citrus aurantium

Origins: Distilled from the blossom of the orange tree.

Aroma: Sweet and floral.

Properties: Antidepressant and antiseptic. It's also reputed to be an aphrodisiac!

Uses: An excellent remedy for stress, skin care, and heart palpitations.

Suggested Blends: Ginger, jasmine, and lavender.

Perfume Note: Middle

Rose Otto

Plant: Rose Otto

Botanical name: Rosa damascena

Origins: Distilled from the fresh rose petals.

Aroma: Sweet, with a hint of vanilla.

Properties: Sedative, antidepressant, and a tonic.

Uses: Rosewater is a popular skin tonic. It is also used to combat menstrual disorders and stress.

Suggested Blends: Geranium, patchouli, chamomile, and frankincense.

Perfume Note: Middle to top

number 8

Sandalwood

Plant: Sandalwood

Botanical name: Santalum album

Origins: Distilled from the tree.

Aroma: Soft, sweet, and woody.

Properties: Antiseptic, anti-inflammatory, and antidepressant.

Uses: Used to treat stress, nausea, colic, and catarrh. It is invaluable for dry or inflamed skin.

Suggested Blends: Patchouli, cedarwood, rose otto, and vetiver.

Perfume Note: Base

Tea Tree

Plant: Tea Tree

Botanical name: Melaleuca alternifolia

Origins: Distilled from the leaves and twigs of the tree.

Aroma: Strongly medicinal.

Properties: Antibiotic, antiseptic, and fungicidal.

Uses: Nature's first aid for fungal infections such as thrush and athlete's foot. An excellent treatment for mouth ulcer's, cold sores, insect bites, and stings.

Suggested Blends: Lavender, spearmint, and geranium.

Perfume Note: Middle

number 10

Diffuse your Dreams

Achieving dreamy room fragrances is easy! Your bedroom will be seductively transformed with a hint of any of the following essential oils, which can all be used with a lamp ring.

A lamp ring is a small, circular ring (metal or ceramic) that sits on top of an upward pointing light bulb. A few drops of your preferred aromatic oil can be dropped on to the ring so that the scent evaporates into the room as it heats up.

You could also try using an electric diffuser. This contains an electric heating element to warm a container for your oils, or by passing air from a fan

through an absorbent pad on
to which you have dropped
some oil.

Alternatively, why don't you make
your own personal diffuser?
Drop some oil on to a pad of
absorbent cotton, place inside a
small tin—make sure the lid has
holes in it. Position on a
radiator to perfume the room.

Tip!

Lamp rings are NOT
recommended for light bulbs
stronger than 60 watts.

Plant: Clove

Botanical name: Eugenia caryophyllata

Origins: Extracted from the flower buds of the clove tree.

Aroma: Slightly bitter and woody.

WARNING!
Do NOT apply directly to skin or inhale via steam applications —best to use as a room scent or fumigant only.

Properties: Antiseptic and anti-rheumatic.

Uses: A classic remedy for toothache, neuralgia, arthritis, and rheumatism. Repels clothes' moths.

Suggested Blends: Rose otto.

Perfume Note: Middle

Clove Bud

Ginger

Plant: Ginger

Botanical name: Zingiber officinalis

Origins: Distilled from the dried rhizomes of the plant.

Aroma: Earthy and spicy.

Properties: Antiseptic and stimulant.

Uses: A wonderful remedy for nausea and for catarrh, congestion, and coughs.

Suggested Blends: Geranium, spearmint, and patchouli.

Perfume Note: Middle/base

Jasmine

WARNING!
Do NOT use
if you are
pregnant.

Plant: Jasmine

Botanical name: Jasminum officinalis

Origins: Extracted from flowers picked after dusk when the oil is at its highest concentration.

Aroma: Heady, exotic, and floral.

Properties: Sedative and antidepressant.

Uses: An excellent tonic for labor pains, premenstrual syndrome, and depression.

Suggested Blends: Chamomile and sandalwood.

Perfume Note: Middle

Plant: Juniper

Botanical name: Juniperus communis

WARNING!
Do NOT use if you are pregnant.

Origins: Extracted from the crushed or dried berries.

Aroma: Fresh and woody.

Properties: Antiseptic and sedative.

Uses: This is beneficial in treating skin, arthritis, and rheumatic conditions.

Suggested Blends: Rose otto and geranium.

Perfume Note: Middle

Lemongrass

Plant: Lemongrass

Botanical name: Cymbopogon citratus

Origins: Extracted from the oriental grass.

Aroma: Sweet and lemony.

Properties: Insecticidal, antiseptic, and a tonic.

Uses: This is good for relieving stress and palpitations. It will also stimulate breast milk in nursing mothers.

Suggested Blends: Geranium, myrrh, palmarosa, and petitgrain.

Perfume Note: Top

Plant: Marjoram

Botanical name: Origanum marjorana

Origins: Extracted from the leaves.

Aroma: Herbaceous, warm, and spicy.

Properties: Digestive, antiseptic, and sedative.

Uses: It lowers blood pressure, eases muscle injuries and sprains, and alleviates insomnia.

Suggested Blends: Juniper and tea tree.

Perfume Note: Middle

Myrrh

Myrrh

WARNING!
Do NOT use
if you are
pregnant.

Plant: Myrrh

Botanical name: Commiphora myrrha

Origins: Extracted from the gum resin of the bark stem.

Aroma: Smoky and balsamic.

Properties: Anti-inflammatory, antiseptic, and sedative.

Uses: This is excellent for healing wounds, and in caring for cracked skin and scars.

Suggested Blends: Cedarwood, frankincense, lemongrass, and patchouli.

Perfume Note: Base

Niaouli

Plant: Niaouli

Botanical name: Melaleuca viridiflora

Origins: Extracted from the young twigs and leaves of the tree.

Aroma: Strong and camphoraceous.

Properties: Antiseptic and digestive.

Uses: For bronchial conditions and insect bites. This is a common ingredient in mouthwashes and toothpastes, and has been used to purify water.

Suggested Blends: Juniper and lavender.

Perfume Note: Middle

Plant: Palmarosa

Botanical name: Cymbopogon martini

Origins: Extracted from the fragrant grass, related to citronella and lemongrass.

Aroma: Geranium-like and sweet.

Properties: Antidepressant and a tonic.

Uses: Will aid nervous exhaustion and stress, and is also used to treat oily skin, acne, and dermatitis.

Suggested Blends: Cedarwood and lavender.

Perfume Note: Middle

Patchouli

Plant: Patchouli

Botanical name: Pogostemon cablin

Origins: Distilled from the soft furry leaves which evoke the fragrance when rubbed.

Aroma: Earthy, musky, and improves with age.

Properties: Stimulant, antidepressant, and a tonic.

Uses: Used to treat dermatitis, abscesses, athlete's foot, nausea, and travel sickness.

Suggested Blends: Geranium, cedarwood, and tea tree.

Perfume Note: Base

Plant: Petitgrain

Botanical name: Citrus aurantium

Origins: Extracted from the leaves and twigs of the same tree which produces neroli oil.

Aroma: Bittersweet

Properties: Digestive and antiseptic.

Uses: This makes an excellent antidepressant, and is recommended for treating acne.

Suggested Blends: Geranium and lavender.

Perfume Note: Top

Petitgrain

Petitgrain

Rosewood

Plant: Rosewood

Botanical name: Aniba rosaeodora

Origins: Extracted from the chipping of the rosewood tree.

Aroma: Soft and woody.

Properties: Boosts the immune system and makes a good antidepressant.

Uses: Use this to rejuvenate mature skin. It also helps to prevent colds and flu.

Suggested Blends: Lavender, jasmine, and tangerine.

Perfume Note: Middle

Rosewood

Rosewood

Plant: Spearmint

Botanical name: Mentha spicata

Origins: Steam distilled from the flower tops.

Aroma: Warm, herbaceous, and mint-scented.

Properties: Digestive and a tonic.

Uses: A good treatment for headaches and nausea, and it is used in the treatment of dermatitis.

Suggested Blends: Tea tree, lavender, and geranium.

Perfume Note: Top

Spearmint

Plant: Tangerine

Botanical name: Citrus reticulata

Origins: Extracted from the peel of the fruit.

Aroma: Fruity and sweet.

Properties: Digestive

Uses: This is good for helping circulation, combating constipation, and diarrhea. It is also used to keep stretch marks at bay.

Suggested Blends: Neroli.

Perfume Note: Top

Tangerine

Tangerine

WARNING!
Do NOT use
if you are
pregnant.

Plant: Thyme

Botanical name: Thymus vulgaris

Origins: Steam distilled from fresh or partly dried leaves and flower tops.

Aroma: Spicy and herbaceous.

Properties: Antiseptic, diuretic, anti-rheumatic, and fungicidal.

Uses: Recommended for respiratory problems including bronchitis and asthma.

Suggested Blends: Marjoram and lavender.

Perfume Note: Middle

Vetiver

Plant: Vetiver

Botanical name: Vetiveria zizanioides

Origins: Related to palmarosa and lemongrass, vetiver is extracted from the dried and chopped (highly fragrant) roots of the grass plant.

Aroma: Earthy and rich—improving with age.

Properties: The "oil of tranquility" is renowned for its calming effect and is a reputed aphrodisiac!

Uses: A popular fixative in the perfume industry.

Suggested Blends: Sandalwood and lavender.

Perfume Note: Base

✓ Always do a patch test before using any essential oil (see page 11).

✓ Always dilute in a carrier oil before applying to your skin.

✓ Always keep essential oil away from your eyes and do not rub your eyes after handling them.

✓ If you are pregnant seek medical advice before using essential oils.

✓ If you are epileptic seek medical advice before using essential oils.